Praise for Psych Murders

"*Psych Murders* is a deeply felt and known work of somatic writing. Stephanie Heit is a writer who does not look away from 'so much unknown,' inhabiting the 'blur' and 'the beauty' in equal measure. How do we write when we're exhausted? Or: How do we survive the book? Heit answers these questions with radical care and visceral acuity, in all weathers."

● BHANU KAPIL ●

"Drawn from the vivid, hallucinatory medical notes Stephanie Heit took during inpatient treatment, *Psych Murders* opens with addresses to the Psych Murderer, a sociopathic bureaucratic persona that feels like an internalized form of the institution: 'You live invisible in the blur of my eye.' The psychiatric institutional setting—with its clinical apparatuses of electroshock treatment—'architected to increase anxiety,' restructures the body and Heit's lines into alternative choreographies, the twitch of synaptic decoherence. The body incorporates the sum total of its treatments and diagnoses—and is a 'DSM-V masterpiece,' which can also be said of the book itself, a devastating and exhilarating read!"

● VIDHU AGGARWAL ●
author of *The Trouble with Humpadori* and *Daughter Isotope*

"*Psych Murders* is a tightly woven and lyrical exposé of the flexibility and failure of language when it remains an accomplice to our collective socialization under ableism. This is necessary and dangerous work, and it is a stunning addition to the crip canon."

• MEG DAY •

author of *Last Psalm at Sea Level*

"Stephanie Heit's *Psych Murders* bears witness to shock treatments, psychiatric wards, and medical interventions. Here suicidal ideation takes the life of an inner murderer, personified. This hybrid lyric memoir pulls no punches. 'I play with pills, pistols, plastics. In my mind. Siren red. Maize and blue of the University Hospital where everyone knows my name.' Harrowing and brave; illuminating and haunting."

• HOA NGUYEN •

author of *A Thousand Times You Lose Your Treasure*

"With tender consideration in the midst of profound psychic pain, Heit guides readers through the journey of psychiatric treatment to confront the 'murderer' in the mind. Suicidal ideation 'crowds out beauty,' but these poems are lucidly crystalline songs of light; not the doctor's interrogative glare but lanterns shining us home."

• ROXANNA BENNETT •
author of *Unmeaningable* and *The Untranslatable I*

"This is a brilliant book of poetry-memoir-witness that crosses many borders and shines a naked and daring light on the horrors of psychic suffering at critical levels beyond the pale of endurance. Stephanie Heit transforms her horrors and scars into a palpable wisdom to benefit others in this magnificent testament to love and survival. She is a starling word- and world-worker and a compassionate, original voice in the wilderness. I bow at her investigative bravery, the loneliness of the journey. 'The brain as abandoned city that just needs some light' is a searing analogy we should all wake up to recognize."

• ANNE WALDMAN •
poet, chancellor emeritus of the Academy of American Poets,
author of *Trickster Feminism*

Made in Michigan Writers Series

GENERAL EDITORS
Michael Delp, Interlochen Center for the Arts
M. L. Liebler, Wayne State University

A complete listing of the books in this series can
be found online at wsupress.wayne.edu

PSYCH MURDERS

Stephanie Heit

WAYNE STATE UNIVERSITY PRESS

DETROIT

ISBN 978-0-8143-4987-8 (paperback)
ISBN 978-0-8143-4988-5 (e-book)

Library of Congress Control Number: 2022933651

Publication of this book was made possible by a generous gift from The Meijer Foundation.

Cover description: The title, *Psych Murders*, appears vertically in large charcoal caps running up and down the page. In the center is a charcoal bipolar neuron with synapses. The nucleus is a black circle with an open mouth and chasm throat in red, perhaps screaming, with pointed white teeth like a shark. On top is the silhouette of a man with a fedora wielding a scythe at the neuron. *Stephanie Heit* is written in red ballpoint cursive on the lower left. The cover is backdropped by cream paper with blue horizontal lines, suggesting large paper sheets used to work on penmanship in school.

On cover: *What I have learned—Bipolar Neuron* by Chanika Svetvilas (2020; charcoal and collage, 36" x 24"). Used by permission of the artist. Cover design by Lindsey Cleworth.

This work is a hybrid memoir poem based on the lived experience of the author while also being an alchemy of memory and imagination. While the places named and/or described may exist, the author has signed multiple forms releasing any medical institutions from any responsibility for harm whatsoever. Resemblances to actual people are accidental. However, suicide and suicidal ideation are very real. Please share with someone when you need care or help. The US system is broken, but there is still support. There is still hope. There are alternatives. Mental health needs to be and can be a community effort.

Wayne State University Press rests on Waawiyaataanong, also referred to as Detroit, the ancestral and contemporary homeland of the Three Fires Confederacy. These sovereign lands were granted by the Ojibwe, Odawa, Potawatomi, and Wyandot Nations, in 1807, through the Treaty of Detroit. Wayne State University Press affirms Indigenous sovereignty and honors all tribes with a connection to Detroit. With our Native neighbors, the press works to advance educational equity and promote a better future for the earth and all people.

Wayne State University Press
Leonard N. Simons Building
4809 Woodward Avenue
Detroit, Michigan 48201–1309

Visit us online at wsupress.wayne.edu

for my parents, Judy & Roger
for your unfailing love, harbor & support

for those who identify with mental health difference,
I honor your experiences & am grateful to you
for bearing witness to some of mine

for psych system survivors, Mad activists,
crip community, disability culture, queer family
& everyone creating new frameworks of care
& imagining a world where we thrive

Contents

To me, the grounds for hope are simply that we don't know what will happen next, and that the unlikely and the unimaginable transpire quite regularly.

—Rebecca Solnit, from "Woolf's Darkness: Embracing the Inexplicable"

Admission Threshold

Strike a match, light a candle. Notice the shadows. We are at the threshold about to enter. This is an act of faith, a step into the unknown, breath practice. Thank you for being in the doorway with me, the safest and strongest part of a structure. Know you can return here if you need to. I'm inviting you into spaces that usually need special keys and diagnosis codes to access: psychiatric locked inpatient units, ECT (electroconvulsive therapy or shock) treatments, bipolar extreme mind states. You will meet my friend and nemesis, Murderer, the gutsy antics of suicidal ideation.

I want you to be safe and cared for in this text that has sharp parts and electricity and murderers. There are places I made on the page for you to rest. To enter. And exit. At will. Not a given in these spaces. Please take whatever time you need to be with these words. This book is not a 72-hour hold, the general time frame of an involuntary psych inpatient admission. This is a shadow text. Let it sing in grunts and incomplete hymns, something scalded. Something lit up and changeable. Matchbook at ready.

■ ■ ■

I spent a lot of time in bed during the period of my life covered in these pages—too exhausted to move, racked with suicidal plans, trying to numb pain with sleep. I had the epigraph to this book written on an index card and taped to the wall where I could see it from my horizontal position. Those words were like a hand reaching out to steady and accompany me through so much unknown. I offer them as a talisman to be with you as you read this book. In the end, it might be useful to know that I'm still here and grateful to be alive:

> *the unlikely and the unimaginable*
> have indeed
> *transpired quite regularly*

Dear Murderer,

Leave me the fuck alone.

You wake me up and put me to sleep with your dangerous temptations: twist the bottle open and empty the pills in my waiting hand. I live with you in my bloodstream jamming neurotransmitters, frontal lobe until you appear like the rational option.

Murderer, I meet your demands: ransom of dates, suicide note, an obituary to lessen the work of those left behind. You live invisible in the blur of my eyes. Success in playing roulette with my breath as I labor inhales and exhales. On my knees, I pray to no god but you.

You infiltrate my daydreams: red splashes the walls, overdose and aspirated vomit guarantee eternal sleep. You drive the taptap of my twilight fingers in their google search for the correct placement of a gun to temple on allhopegone. com. My clinical notes dictate: *extremely suicidal, this patient's baseline.*

You crowd out beauty. The water that used to shape me into driftwood and limbs articulate. You make emptiness an acquired aesthetic. Force me to stomach it daily. Trade pain for nothing. Make yourself an easy choice I don't execute. Murderer, you don't let up. Even when I'm locked up under constant observation, you hover.

I am a soldier in training for your death army too scared of you to enlist. We won't find a compromise. Pulse. No pulse. For now, I negotiate dates and procrastinate our meeting. Sooner or later. You win. You always win.

Yours truly.

WAITING BAY

Rows of beds with bodies wheeled down from the top floor inpatient unit to the basement. Hospital gowned bodies to be moved, turned, tended as diagnosis codes. IVs attached to veins located and plumbed. Wristband particulars. Blood pressure cuff velcroed around right ankle. Sticky leads attached to chest. Beeping sounds from the curtained-off room we wait to enter. Fear wipes out any smells. Dry mouth taste from anesthesia fast and panic.

No comfort of walls. Head to foot we are lined up in symmetry—semblance of order. Perhaps the queue to cross Styx. My coins ready, though the metal may prove problematic with electric current. Jewelry removed, which amounted to my watch. Exception for wedding rings surgically taped to refute the charge. Hetero privilege. The space pants out of its mouth—almost hyperventilates dried up from lack of liquid, cringes at what it holds.

These bodies prepared for electrocution. Waivers signed. MRIs complete. Physicals. The ECT memory tests. 1–10 scale. Hamilton Depression Rating Scale. Chest monitors applied. The space didn't want this. It was basement. Thoroughfare not adept for this much gravity. These bodies shuttled. Broken. Beyond normal repair routes. The space an absence of smell. Gap between antiseptic and betadine. A smell that stopped caring about being a smell. No ambition to register.

Klonopin before I get here. Accumulation of treatments, my mind picks a fear focus: waking up in the middle. A fellow inpatient elder remembers this happening in the late 60s in Ford Hospital. Another fear focus: bathroom. I needed to go. *You're next in the shock drive-thru. Don't worry.* I woke to urine-soaked sheets, urine film my body harbored the four hour ride home. Subsequent sessions, multiple awkward bathroom trips in anticipation. Transfer the IV drip to mobile steel stand, non-slip socks placed on my feet, journey

around the corner with hospital gown bare dignity cover.

Waiting space

architected to increase anxiety. No piped-in music. No peony photograph-lined walls. No paint colors picked for uplifting properties. This is basement: fluorescent lit, packed with gurneys of hopeless. Occasional rush of *make way* as a human hooked to machines and entourage of surgical-gowned people run through.

Early days I didn't need a line. They put a PICC in my right AC while I was under during the first ECT. Rubber tube sticking out of me. Hybrid. Protagonist in my own speculative fiction. When I left inpatient, my mom flushed it twice daily. Inside to outside monitored and cleaned. Two second hook up to saline. Ready. And wait.

My body fills with the sea.

The medical world waited over a decade to do this. ECT proposed during a hospitalization when I was 27. Three doctors concurred. I'd been in a therapy group with a recent Johns Hopkins ECT graduate. She sat barely speaking with a folder of labeled pictures to remind her of her life. The doctor didn't like my no. Saw it as a symptom rather than a choice. He required me to watch an outdated VHS tape documenting a shock treatment from the 70s. The nurse assigned to document my compliance was horrified.

Pincushion trial. Teaching hospital. After both residents have a go (repeat this every session) they get the nurse from another department, vein whisperer, who swoops in and taps me like a hypersensitive woodpecker finds critters in a tree trunk. She gets it, makes sure the IV flows. This time in the wrist. Fragile thin. I wait with a girl next to me from the children's unit. Just outline. Her features almost not. Wish to be invisible and ultimate desire to disappear nearly realized. We breathe the hospital basement air, antiseptic and stale, more carbon dioxide than oxygen. Not enough inhales.

Jackhammer therapy. Yet another last ditch option before ECT. *Good candidate*, they said. Boys with their toys. A new machine must be used. Daily. Forty minutes. I don't remember much. A kind woman my mom and I stayed with, name forgotten. The rest is anecdotal. The Friday dessert at the Crazy Wisdom Tea Room to celebrate another five-day-my-brain-as-construction-site done. Walks at Gallup Park in silence or one-sided conversation. *Transcranial Magnetic Stimulation*. I don't remember any effects. Just the sound and the pain. And the long computer questionnaire I had to fill out every week to quantify shitty on a 1–10 scale.

A bay as if we are sheltered, waiting to sail out into unruly ocean. Hull and masts serviced, ready. We will not see open water today. Unless underanesthesia visions—brain free from what brings us to steel beds to this hail mary procedure. One bay to the other side, another bay. Anchored by tubes and lost will. After enough of these crossings you forget

$\qquad\qquad\qquad\qquad\qquad\qquad$ how to swim.

$\qquad$ Forget

$\qquad\qquad\qquad$ your tokens.
$\qquad\qquad\qquad\qquad$ Lose any sense

$\qquad\qquad$ of direction.

Jigsaw puzzle where I can't match the corners. Box lost with the picture. Hard to ask for a piece when I don't know it's missing. Chance operation starts with *do you remember when . . . ?* Snag free brain. I'm a vulnerable narrative. Who am I and what have I done? Breath catches. Somatic wisdom: the body remembers. When the body goes AWOL normal rules don't apply.

Dear Brain,

I'm sorry.

I remember when Whitecoat told me I'd have a new brain after this, like it was a present. I felt sadness even in my apathetic stupor. I liked my original brain. This new one fails me, betrays its injuries daily as I navigate my city only with Siri's aid. It acts more colander than container.

CAN
YOU
THINK
ABOUT
THE
FUTURE?

The Shock Machine: Neuromodulation Master

I make brains quake. Bodies rupture. Bones break. In the old days before anesthesia and muscle relaxants. Now it's passive city while I charge through dead end streets, *this way only* signs going the wrong direction. Ordinary day of sizzle. Electrons vibrate, a contagious undertaking. I leave indelible marks. The aftermath memory loss, pianists who forget how to play, loved ones now strangers, that sort of thing. My charges are almost all women. And the ones hitting the go button, men. I'm neutral. A funny thing for a conductor to say but my orchestra plays the indifferent sonata. *Don't kill the messenger* is my motto. I go where directed. I'm held in the shaky hands of shock virgin residents. My main contact is with the temple and top of head of my charges. I don't get attached, even though some of them return three times a week. My job is to induce the juice, not to track my electrical impact. I leave that to Whitecoats. There is a movement

to ban me. Afraid of my power, no doubt.
Or the fact I'm not FDA approved. I buzz
my electroconvulsive melody, staccato
and consistent at 70–150 volts for 0.1–0.5
seconds. I turn that excitable brain tissue
on, light bulbs aflicker in so much dark.

Procedure Details

the seizure lasted minutes
Adequate

how many inhales and exhales does it take
No Post Procedure Agitation
to turn over time
ECT device:
watch mechanics to create future
in flutters temporal and pulsing
Thymatron or MECTA

to tick down language
increments *s motor 62*
make a tempo I can curve *s*
EEG 75

the past oil slicks
to open water
its own neuroplastic sun
dial lubricates shadows
illuminates the digits

but here is disappearance
Unless stated otherwise,
sensation of drowning
for this procedure the EBL is zero
but drowning in a calm way
no urgency to reach
surface
grab
air

waterboarding for the brain
Electrode Placement: Bilateral
hijack neural pathways
injure tissue so the healing
might alter the before
see flow sheet

one moment bleeds into every

like monarch wings that keep vibrating
glottis at back of throat
good induction
each word infused
unable to recall 3 of the 5

initial words during delayed recall
the joke is memory loss
only able to name 7 words
that begin with the letter "S" within a minute
benevolence in not remembering

breathe water call it quenching thirst

if I put enough words down
I was present for the entire procedure
Electronically signed by _____ *MD/13530*
a balm to slather all the pockmarks
I don't know how to fill
Patient is sad in affect with mild preservation of reactivity

I tried not to be electric
The patient has been reluctant
to consider ECT due to significant trepidation and anxiety
not to be their voltage conductor
See the past medical history for details
not horizontal and asleep

tolerated procedure well

Tell yourself this is ok. You are Whitecoat messiah do-gooding into oblivion. Read the stats and only believe the success figures. Erase the possibility of harm from your conscience with evidence-based congratulatory devices. Anesthetize doubt. Make a propaganda video with reassuring clips from patients and family. Forget the gowned bodies are human. Taste power. Don't think about how you have no idea how this works. Strengthen your faith in electricity. The brain as abandoned city that just needs some light.

Six months out the creak of the house sets my amygdala on fire. Night terrors. High startle response. ECT events replay over and over in my head. Loops I don't escape. Do no harm. And we all fail.

I minimize the memory loss by telling myself the dead have no memory.

I ask them to be murderers. Ask them to add more anesthesia. I know it's a tricky business, that it is easy to make a mistake. Make a mistake, I plead. Please, I beg. This would be kind. They interrupt my talking with oxygen over my face and instructions to breathe deeply. Whitecoat says I will feel better after this. It is number ___. I can't remember what number it is. Somewhere between 5 and 25, probably.

I wake up after.
I don't feel better.
Start planning.
Again.

The Murderer: 401K

People ask how I keep up my impeccable record. I'd like to say persistence, dedication, passion, those trademark American work ethic values. But really, it's the easiest job ever. I was made for this. Maybe I should get a better PR agent. Make this look tough: highlight my intensive workout regimen, daily target practice, psychological studies of my clients so I know their tics. I could charge more but figure a life is enough. Some lives are worth more than others, but it balances out in the end. With such high demand and escalating suicide rates, I've played with the idea of expanding: employees, increased revenue, wider service offerings. But I prefer the control of my one-man-murderer band. I can be selective and only take the difficult cases, leave the rest to the amateurs (luring a person in an extreme mind state to jump off a bridge is below me, pardon the pun). I've thought about retirement. Kick back in the La-Z-Boy a bit more. Take a beach holiday that doesn't involve rocks in pockets, boat "accidents," or unexplained rip currents. Some work is for life, in my case death, and there is no retirement package from who you are.

WHAT BRINGS YOU PLEASURE?

Murderer hangs out with me 24/7. Actually, there is a much needed reprieve with sleep. 10 hours. Then 12. Then 14. Afternoon arrives. My Murderer is there as soon as I wake up. Surprises me at my Monday night yoga class when I'm in shavasana trying to bliss out. Lies next to me. Says: *corpse pose is my favorite.* Says: *go home and kill yourself.*

Murderer shows up uninvited at my Spanish group to announce that I won't be there next week. It is a full time job trying to stay alive and trying to get dead at the same time. He traces my every move, always has me within sightlines, prepared and trigger ready, non-stop threat until the desire to get rid of his cadaver breath on my neck becomes more urgent than a death toll. The tension of when Murderer will find me unprepared and how he will kill me builds until any action would be release.

Tired of looking over my shoulder, tracking Murderer's movements, measuring his strength, gauging when to call for help. Days then months then years of this dead end relationship. Both of us stuck and unhappy. Unable to call it quits.

Exhausted to the point of death fantasies. I walk towards his welcoming arms. My Murderer embraces me. Leads me in a slow dance. I match his tempo, a rhythm to coax me to the other side. I reach my foot over the line. Sense the freefall beyond, the irreversibility of a step too far. Feel Murderer's breath on my neck, my pulse emptying.

I get scared. I make the calls, wait the wait, explain again to a psych ER resident my unusual med cocktail, humor the questions, and eventually arrive on the unit. When I enter, Murderer lets me out of his crosshairs. I sink under the comfort of hospital white.

(in)voluntary

bleach seductress / call it hypnotism / locked door
luxury / food delivered in ready-to-eat portions
/ jello! / swish of carts / all the touches / blood
pressure cuff / pulse monitor / thermometer /
doctors / tidy boxes / if you fit the criteria / which
I do! / pill & needle zombie elixirs / magnetism of
suicide / precaution questions / oh to be a number
on a 1–10 scale! / walls sing lullabies / no, that is
not screaming / notice the softness / no sharps here
/ right angles / lose their rightness / white intake
sheet raised / I give myself up

Forecast

I lose the concept of weather. Forehead presses unbreakable glass. Instances of long term memory loss are rare and statistically insignificant. Stand waist deep in ocean riptides & undertow. What is your job? Staying alive. What does that look like? CV of psychiatric hospitalizations. Translate my inner laboratory into DSM. Touchdown & taken. Project life. I hesitate in traces. Adrenalin shuttle. Gulp the future. Temptation to bleach this history. Signposts in sorrow & paperwork usurped signature. Look for it in corridors antiseptic & narrowing. I lose my breath. Wall of anesthesia ghosts through. Left hand where the IV leaves its mark. Inhale the bardo. Pickaxe & night. Double locked doors. Walls thick. Windows transparent when nothing else is.

The doors are locked, windows unbreakable and sealed shut. I don't add Murderer to my guest list. There is sanctuary. His constant surveillance substituted with scales of 1 to 10; percentages of food eaten, hours slept; check marks for bowel movements and showers; blood pressure reads; and privileges based on compliance. Stop gaps: codes, alarms on the tops of doors, inventories of sharps, locks on med cart, plastic forks and spoons, no knives, no shoelaces, no belts, no spiral ring journals. No ammunition for my Murderer unless he gets creative. He tries to slip into my get-ready-for-bed routine. Launches a *Just Do It* ad inside my head to the speed of my toothbrush. Or first thing in the morning, *notice the electrical cords in the dayroom*, when the brand new day is not what I ordered on the breakfast menu.

Throw a Pill at It

Objectified patient stands in the corner while a flock of Whitecoats, including fledglings with undeveloped aim, hurls pills at it. Objectified patient receives a unique cocktail throw (or throws, as it takes a college try) dependent on its personality cluster traits and, of course, genetic predisposition(s). Blue. Yellow. Pink. Triangle. Ellipse. Circle. Capsules burst upon impact—micro yellow and green balls hop on hygienically cleaned linoleum. The pill arsenal—SSRIs, antipsychotics, benzos, stabilizers, stimulants—soars through the air like psychotropic confetti. Objectified patient receives the impact with arms raised skyward in the assumed position. Its face, impartial and aloof, matches the morning assessment: *flat affect, apathy 10*. Whitecoats try to appear professional: stern man faces regardless of gender, but today, like so many days, all men. They take aim. Flick the pills where they will do the most good. Hope for the best. Start wrist workouts at lunch to combat carpal tunnel and gain technique. Under the white coats so highly prized for their authoritative fashion and whiteness in spite of this bloody work (the goal is to break its

skin), under the name tag MD loud and proud—
their hearts collectively lub dub at a quickened
pace. Thrill of the gamble, the it in the corner,
all those neurotransmitters and the crapshoot
odds of the flick-it skills of the flock. Objectified
patient turns clockwise, meat on a skewer, pelted
on every side. It knows the schedule. Dinner
soon. It will receive a percentage for the amount
of food it eats, smiley or sad face for the bowel
movements it does or doesn't make, check mark
for the shower it takes. It will be questioned to
test its desire to live, level of hope, physical
safety. Whitecoats research evidence-based-
trajectory strategies: adjust pill arc, flight time,
point of contact. Wonder what is wrong with it
when it doesn't get better in these optimal
circumstances.

They never ask the
       flight patterns of
            its dreams.

TREATMENT ROOM

Drive-thru fast. Curtain pulled. Bed head
hinged horizontal. Doctor in the corner in
white. Anesthesiologist out of sight behind
my head. I interrupt the oxygen mask, ask
for names. Before I am ready they push
sleep,

                              push their batons
on both my temples, hit on.

Whoosh sound

like awareness sucked
with a giant vacuum cleaner from inside
my head when in reality awareness numbed
from muscle relaxants administered so
I become a noodle immune to seizure.
Twitches subdued. Beyond apathy. Course
of energy through my system. Blaze through
channels. Reboot the computer with a
new background color. My body inert,
ambivalent in white gown, covered in white
blanket but for my right foot cuffed off
flutter, toe digits wave farewell to control,
spastic tempo hits the bridge, reverberates
until the power is cut. The rest of my body
a still point, enforced rest.

Oxygen at ready in case
my lungs.   Crash cart in case
my heart. Brain shaken like a scared animal
shakes off fear. Swollen. Injured. Big in my
head. Repercussions invadethemomentthe
nextmomentrepetitionofmomentsthen
the subtraction   of   moments   seized
loose.

Lost.

Going out goes hard. The meds burn in. *Shitshitshit* under my breath under the oxygen mask. They push more. Get her out. Get sleep. Get on with it. Background fear that the vein will give, anesthesia fail: I'll wake up being electrocuted. The mental health worker grabs my hand. She rubs my forearm firmly—a distract sensation from the burning. Touch, usually a side effect of blood pressure cuff placement, pulse monitor, thermometer. Implements rather than skin. This is the only instance I remember someone holding my hand out of kindness. *Thank you D.*

Extra drugs reverse the anti-anxiety drugs that are also anti-seizure drugs. They want a good seizure. To control lightning, the strike and the results. Medieval medicine. Whitecoats are believers or sadists. Burden of ECT stigma they work to bust. Nurse Ratched stereotypes. They make their points sharp: *safe, effective, rare long term memory loss*. Validate the unknown like afterlife guarantees.

Dear Doctor,

Dear God,

I don't remember the first treatment. I know I was inpatient with a blue sticky note *NPO* on the outside of my door so the staff knew no water or food. I doubt I slept much the night before. Probably scared. Or perhaps so apathetic I didn't care. The room surprised me. Makeshift. Pop up. Box of volts in the corner. Electrical outlet of course. Anesthesiologist crammed in the rear. Monitors. A curtain more decorative than functional. Shit colored. Tile floor so the gurney could wheel fast in the event of an emergency. I am inside the event of an emergency. The doctor in white (I picture blood splotches for every ECT administered, each brain wave distorted—now he is red) probably reviews the procedure, slows the pace by a beat. Then sleep. Curtain over my eyes. But before, promises of *Better.* More fortune teller than MD. More crapshoot superstition than science.

I refused this space.

My refusal seen
as a desire to die—*if you are already going
to die, why not try this treatment that could save
your life?* Shock my brain and body. Scramble
memory. Add trauma to tissue as agency for
good. This goes against everything I know
to be true as a dancer. My body intelligence,
honed awareness. This is a nonsensical
violent enterprise. To pretend electricity
leaves no trace. To pretend my body is not
me. To divorce myself from consciousness
and go with a method that in the early days
was heralded as replacement lobotomy.

Think about doughnuts
is the send off. Because he really likes
doughnuts, and this is what he would want
to anesthesia ponder. The phrase adds a
surrealist edge, potentially cruel as none of
us—the to-be-shocked ones—have eaten
since the night before.

Pick out a good dream
is its eventual replacement. Go nowhere,
dream nothing would be my reality. Every
under feels like death practice. I ask them
to keep me there.

Like tides, patients roll in and out. Series of
birthdates. Names. Little gender variance.
Keep with history. Not much space. An inlet
appears protected but steep cliff,
unstable rocks. Not permanent. Psychiatry
rents out this room (technically three walls
and flimsy hardly private curtain) for their
morning high tide. Five days a week. Full
moon pull. The waters in our bodies vibrate.
Landslide. Brain fried. Next.

I rest with all the blank spaces, neurotransmitter blips, gum eraser track marks. History as improvisation. Document gone through the shredder. Is it worth the effort to reassemble? Fluff and dust the years. Insert myself. They say it will come back. Like answering the doorbell to a character who enters with host of details and their name/connection. This is my reeducation. Don't worry about the holes. The hard part being no one else sees them so they share histories with me I don't remember.

Dear Right Foot,

I'm grateful you got to dance it out. Embody flutter and seize. Sense yourself in time and space. Keep the beat to an unfortunate tune, the staccato section of the ECT marching band. Team Whitecoat. Team hopeless. Win uncertain. Rules unknown. Equipment not FDA approved. My right foot invents new time signatures. Shakes its digits in the sterile air. The most movement folks with catatonia experience all week. I no longer dance or sing and have all but stopped talking. But my foot launches into soliloquy.

SPELL

WORLD

BACKWARD

Window   Dressing

Murderer is undefined. I close the curtains against him so there is no crack for the unexpected. Always dress in socks then underwear, shirt then pants. Tend the daytime hours and hurry the night into abeyance. I monitor the dark, take his pulse with quickened breath, nervous system primed. Hypervigilance to keep the outside from taking root. The apple tree with its ominous shadow, arms clawed and eager. Before amnio and womb where she died, my sister left her essence to become part of me. I live liminal, sensitive to the music beyond the underpinnings of exits, the seductive gasp of nowhere. My insides weeded to make space for her light. I impose Martial Law on my single digit self. Or Murderer does. Patrols the edges of sleep. I sit on the stair landing, peek below to my parents' voices. I don't tell them I'm scared. Don't mention him. Fear that tastes like Flintstones vitamins, soundtrack of *Jaws*. Closets shut tight to keep the corners clear. I check my pulse, make sure we still beat. She and I, pulse in two. I live in both: the darkness wants me more.

Rehearsal

Murderer held the mirror hostage. I danced full out. Long limbs still growing, finding their unique rhythm, wingspan. I dodged his glare. Reveled in movement. Flowed through space with ease. Still, he'd catch me unawares and pull apart the across-the-floor sequence like a predator locating gristle on a kill. I'd turn away stone-faced, try again. I succeeded in avoiding him for the most part. Until I didn't. Murderer got inside. Found the weak points and grapevined over them. Bikini class to teach me how to hate my body. Made me into a soldier for his war: beat yourself up more than anyone else ever could. But I outdanced him. Worked hard. Spite. Resilience. Determination. Passion. I didn't have a chance. Part of his training was to spot predisposition. Potential. Easy target. Game plan: take away the one thing I loved.

Yours truly,

A limbic dream, reptilian longevity liable to outlast me. I try to conjure you:

safety on, adrenalin ready, amnesia grace.

Yours is a face I forget.

I could blame it on poor recall.

But you are wallpaper, backdrop to the city I left, geographically

inconsequential. A construct pillar and pith broken.

I built that city rock and quake with electricity tremor.   You, the mayor,

executive orders at ready to strain the constraints, make me targeted,

easy bait for your wipe-out games.   And the undertow,

high tide always.

Escape routes negligible but my mind, trick seamstress, hemmed me pickle.

This wait game stale as hyperventilation.   You liked me raw,

                myelin sheath shaved filigree rampant.

      Duet to the tune of a panic attack with a cappella hospital ward

walls for the coda.

      You promised and broke me pretty.

      Underground   tunnel to the lowest rung.

Not bravery, desperation of the body through a needle eye you can't miss.

Or that hurtle into space, let's go!   House lights fade to black,

           come up

     empty

.

The navigational chip in my head got knocked. I need instructions for which way to turn at the end of the driveway. Can't locate the bathroom in the yoga studio. Forget where my best friend lives. Even after a year, I need the vigilance of Google Map Woman to make it to the location of my weekly Spanish group. I don't hold the city grid in my body—topographical disorientation. The place cells in my hippocampus lost. Wayfinder skills nonexistent. I live in a micro-directional landscape with room for where I am and not for where I am going. I don't like driving with people since I need full concentration to get from A to B and get embarrassed when I don't know how to get to B, C, D. When I say I don't know where Gallup Park is and the person gives cross streets and the school nearby, or even worse, the compass-oriented clan tell me it's on the southeast side of town on the north side of the street, I learn to nod and say *yes, yes I do know where that is* since those navigational types take *I don't know* as a challenge and don't give up until I am the star on the map

you are here.

Sleep touches me, leaves smears like snail tracks I wipe off throughout the day. Web spun silky trap I can't shake. The GPS miscalculates and I end in the wrong life.

This is someone else's thread needling my larynx. I speak words not my dictionary. Vocabulary of doubt and down. Parlance of silence. The blank pools at sleep's bottom. Escape mechanism snooze. Turn the day over. Flip the sun to the other side. This night chest ridden and haunt.

I don't remember that picture

body with memories inscribed in other tongues
throat of pockets to keep language from
falling take these zippers un &
zip this is doing a crested action
traces ashy memory *me not me*
I am pink gum eraser the mouthguard positioned
histories gone no aftertaste
tell me about the border crossing
the stamp on my palm faded
where the anesthesia went in before
soundproof panels spaghetti in the brain

tell me the seizure of here to there
the tremble in the going

anything I can touch I could be

                                             steel pillar with cracks
                                             corner held up by light blue

walls

                                             piano pedals & sleek lines
                                             wishlist of crossed out verbs

& fly

                                             jangle skeleton on a ferry
                                             undertow & over
                                             the deep parts where sharks

mate

                                             this body cross-legged &

then gone

                                             buzz of fluorescence

somewhere, future

I fell outside of me

floorboard vibrations   right foot flutter seizure   eyes closed softness
the wall moves closer
my ankle cracks
thoughts aloud thoughts loud
she is awake   I am the waker   I can't stop
this is not supportive
other bodies   sometimes corners   the room creates more
darkness has a smell
there is sticky in her breath that won't come out
enclosed parts lodged
she trains my mind to stay and it goes
wind knocked out as the wall catches
markers in my blood
controlled then   I hear them   breathing
she licks the wall and it tastes
there are certain balances
do not say *broken*
the stitches a fiber art experiment
her feet sleepdance
cushion raft   blue grades   piano sheen
I navigate by sound magnified through muscle

DO YOU HAVE A SPECIFIC PLAN?

Secondary Crime Scene

The first ten pages blur.

      Only traces:

                        articles,   nouns.

                                          If you had the verbs.

                          Run:

                                  verb or

                                  noun?

Call this blank space. Inside your head failure of gray matter. Let go instead of retain. Google *memory loss*. List of possible causes includes ECT and bipolar disorder.

The first ten pages. A room you never entered but are expected to know contents, interior design, and location in the building.

You are ten pages from the beginning.

> Password to Netflix account.
> Year you finished grad school.
> Directions home.
> Why you love someone.
> Who that person is.

They occupy dreamspace. Later in the cycle before you awake. The stuff you lose. Residual feeling of having fought, twisted sheets, sweat, but you have no idea what happened.

You need those ten pages to survive.

> What are your strategies?
> Will you ask people for help?
> Tie red threads around your fingers?
> Ingest ginkgo leaves?
>
> How will you live with the empty white business-sized security envelopes filed away in your head?

You could make up those ten pages.

Create a new beginning.
Turn the page.
Hands shaky.
Memory confidence at low.

Your sequence includes clearing your throat, an extension of a "tip of
the tongue" moment, backward movements of the arms and legs (reverse
crawl for swimmers, wheelbarrow rolls for the land-based). Search
for seed moments that will bring a page back. You get used to that
unanchored feel. The photos of yourself in landscapes and with groups of
people you don't recognize.

Make your life around the ten pages.

Yellow crime scene tape surrounds the missing.
Another murder unsolved.

Not tip of the tongue loss
    but snow that covers the landscape and you can no longer find your car.

Words like taxidermy butterflies, carefully placed pins and containers preserve once flap once flight once migration. They shake themselves loose, recirculate in dreams that turn nightmare with current running through and power all in the wrong hands. Mine pinned immobile by my sides. I wake sweaty and dry mouthed. Up for air from a world that has none. I herd words into corrals. Create new forms to hold what my body cannot. Wonder if the page is substantial enough. Worry it with my pen. Will it give? Evaporate like memories no longer mine. I write on loose leaf paper. Unattached. Turned sideways the shape of the Post Anesthesia Care Unit. When a place holds the material. And it's you.

Those years burned me   blazon and ash. I sift wreckage for remnants. Shiny things above the melting point. They say fertile, new growth after. But for a long time, scar. An opening that wouldn't make itself presentable. Agape and drooly. Smell of past due and deliver me someplace else already. I dressed it up real nice. Three letter rearranged acronym, different comfort.

ECT Autocorrected to ETC.

Words difficult to hold in the mouth. Charged. Like biting into a live animal. Slithery cries. Beg to be released. Spit it out. Let the thing live independent. Change consonant order. Disengage from heartbeat quicken and hand quake. Push to the edge. Snails circumnavigate the glass, clean. Let them be clean. Not the dint and tarry of labor. Words that have worked too hard. To mean. To bite. To jar. To hook strings of thought to jugulars then bleed. They leave their shadows.

Synonyms with less
pizzazz deflect the
zing. Still bitter, still
stench. Some days
they advance. Take the
body hostage. Reign
with serif feet and
bold cursory.
Overtaken. Tweezers
debride them from
your skin. Bone deep
ones past viscera
vibrate you. Get
marrow. Get
mainlined until you
taste their spice.
Dilute with
ambivalence and amnesia.
Pretend you
are not this alphabet.

I didn't expect the zoo. The gawkers: *Really?* The extinctionists: *They don't do that anymore. Do they?* The speciests: *My grandmother, cousin, friend of a friend had that done.* And the deflectors: *Well, you seem just fine now.*

Mad Flora and Fauna Catalog: Turtle

Turtle is the depression animal. Or rather this was the animal I aligned with
when I was finding my way forward or who knows in what direction, some
compass dislocated from a ship long splattered in the ocean. A wreck of
suicidal ideation and concrete planning I never thought I'd find my way away
from alive. This is turtle. The slow movement. Middle ground. Ability to
pull into a home a shell or my own skin. A limbic striated reach toward the
beach that gave me shore and light. Steady. No acrobatic feats. Simply alive.
Pull and extend. A bit of push, but not too much, because I'm tired.

The Classifieds: Bipolar Girls on a Manic High are my Addiction

look for the bipolar girls sexy if you can get them
manic god-like confidence and unlimited energy
till they hum rubbing on streetpoles pure libido
oozing out crotches a slippery invitation those
bipolar chicks will surprise you stripping off
clothes without an invitation not even caring what
your name is just that you are fuck ready bipolar
chick like an animal randy in heat hit that if you
can if you are brave enough to mess with crazy

Mad Flora and Fauna Catalog: Hyena

Hyena is the manic animal. Famished fanged with a haunted look. Nocturnal prowl on the edges of other worlds. Cursorial like my mind. Race to kill with the teeth. Rip prey to pieces. Steal. Drive. Run. Cuts on my arm to release the pressure. Red of inside meets outside. *You look like a ghost* my mother said in the hospital after I'd had my stomach lavaged. Hyena. A spirit. Looks sideways. Part dog part cat part unnameable. Not trustworthy. Laughing at myself.

Solar Eclipse

when light comes off me, radiance that
competes with the sun, when words appear
from unknown sources, an expanded
vocabulary beyond my regular capacity,
when biology ticks faster & sleep is an
unnecessary bedmate when I'm going & it
doesn't matter where but there are sparks
& electrical synapse fires I don't want to put
out *burn baby! I take all the oxygen in the room*
when I need less food but grow taller when
my body shimmers due to high vibration
when my hands don't know stillness & my
brain is ferris wheel with tickets for sale
& I can't get off I'm all alone & ideas keep
on & slowly the tides rise & I'm flooded
& freak for an island but I drown & I've
done this enough I'm prepared to activate
nightvision, initiate suicide watch, sleep
deep in the belly of darkness, pull it long
into my lungs like a hit that leaves me flat
& I keep breathing knowing some day this
darkness will keep me

Out of range Murderer's quick sights fail.

He bets on tomorrow, but it doesn't come.

Not now.

Still not.

Now.

Not yet.

RECOVERY BAY

Slow return to sensation   .

Bleached white sheets scratch. Material's memory of the multiple other patients they've touched. Some discharged. Some dead. I wonder the threshold for bodily fluids—when too much red retires them. Bed side rails up to keep gravity at bay. This month the psych unit won the demerit for most falls. I wake curled fetal banked by pillows. Sound returns as it left,
          low whoosh

                    like distant sea. Slur of noise enunciates as a face in my face:

Stephanie, do you know where you are?

I could order the hospital records for accuracy, but I know there would be vomit. I know there was a headache of seismic proportions. Brain shaken like a tambourine. Swell. Blood rushes to the injury. Revision: not *injury*—*therapeutic site*. This is healing. I spend the day to night sleeping off the anesthesia. The sedation cocktail is altered two days later at the next session to include *toradol* to lessen the head pain. That night or another night—some night of my many inpatient nights—TV in the patient rec room tuned to *One Flew Over the Cuckoo's Nest*.

I maintained my no for over a decade. No ECT. No hospitals. My health relied on outpatient care, an intense med and well-being regimen, and staying away from psychiatric institutions. No locked doors. No new diagnosis codes. I never imagined it would get so bad I'd sign the line. I'd submit to their rigors. I'd turn my body over until it was no longer my body. I'd want out so bad I'd say yes. They saw hope when my consent was giving up. Do whatever you want because I don't care anymore, I don't have energy to fight you, I don't exist. Run out of options and alternatives. Show me your back pocket coins. Your voltage. Your seizure illusions.

Passed out bodies return from the room red, elevated blood pressures, facial twitches, mouthguards stick out lips until the nurses remove them. Check vitals. Make sure there is still breath and heart. Hold plastic containers to catch vomit. The involuntary urine and shit during a seizure will be dealt with later. Oxygen masks, paddles on standby. Before we return to the top floor, we must pass orientation tests:

Stephanie, you are waking up from ECT.
You are in the University Hospital.
Can you tell me your name?
Can you tell me where you are?

I swam. Too deep to return to the name on my wristband. The touch on my shoulder saying you are done. I was under, past where light reaches, perpetual dark no luminescent creatures to beam a glimpse of surroundings. Past synapse. A pseudo death. A nothing realm. They call me back. To mark their checklist of vitals. Count me among the accounted. Elevator up into a world I can't breathe. Can't concentrate. Forget my reasons. Maze to navigate morning. And I want the under. To stay below. For the machines to stop. Lines like a midnight horizon.

I don't remember waking up. Don't remember the questions, the vital checks. Don't remember curling up fetal style. Don't remember the elevator ride up to the 9th floor. Don't remember putting on my clothes. The see-you-in-3-days niceties with the ECT staff. Don't my dad pushing the wheelchair. Don't the hospital cafeteria. Don't the checkout line and the pity looks. Don't the 4 hour drive home. Don't the silence.

Hope became a location. A hallowed facility with the victors, hail to Whitecoats with research funding. The city became sanctuary or expedition, where I travelled to find answers. I thought they'd figure out the code. No lack of rigor. But my body didn't respond the way the data predicted. They couldn't find me in databases or their empirical knowledge.

Shored up. Ample nausea drugs, pain killers, ice water in styrofoam cups with straws. Yes, an extra pillow. I mostly don't remember this part. In my chart mark *unreliable narrator*. Sleep. Wake. I take in this side of the room from the other. Like shoreline cartography easier to make out with distance. In the elevator I wake up, ask if it is over. *You woke up in the recovery bay and answered orientation questions; it is a safety measure.* I wonder what part of me responded. Drift back to sleep. Hard sleep. Like my head pressed underwater in the deep until I hit bottom.

I investigate what my body did. See a program on ECT with a scene at the University with one of the Whitecoats. I can't look away. Whitecoat places his hand on her foot while she is seizing (notice the pronouns, they rarely change). My cells rally screaming, *Don't touch her.* I want to know what happened to my body while I was away. Who touched me. What pressure. Where. During the seizure what did my face do. *Homeland* Claire Danes ECT scene. I look away. But glance at the TV before it is over. I replace my face with her squinched one, arched neck.

I'm left at the ECT emergency exit. Last shock done. No one to guide me through the next days, then months, then years. Whitecoat denial of memory loss. Traumatic Brain Injury. Damage. No rehab or support groups for what does not happen. Open sea.

ARE
YOU
SAFE?

The big claim of support groups is the YOU ARE NOT ALONE diatribe. I know I'm not alone. I have Murderer stalking my every move. I can't say he keeps me company or tells me bedtime stories. He never commiserates or compares histories with me. But I'm never alone. He isn't the type to attend these support groups. Works solo and doesn't like talking about his job, which tends to be frowned upon with the killing and all.

I play with pills, pistols, plastics. In my mind. Siren red. Maize and blue of the University Hospital where everyone knows my name.

Chronic

Chronic sounds like forever. Persistent forever. With a twang to the way the "ic" sticks in the throat. Almost guttural. Starts out ok. Chron, like chronological, that domino effect, out of control falling because gravity exists. But the ending turns. I am stuck with Chronic the rest of my life. Better than Terminal unless it refers to airports. Though at least with Terminal there is beginning, middle, end. Chronic is middle with no way out. Unpredictable. Dormant waiting to awaken and execute my plans and passions in Russian roulette. I live wishing Chronic would grow some balls and kill me. I suppose you want a clearer profile: aftershave preference, cigarette brand, hours spent at the shooting range, recreational activities not involving guns, favorite dinner. This isn't safe. Because it changes. Murderer's presence is vague. Takes my breath. Plays it fast. Plays it slow. Plays. Hands tight around my heart. Takes my body. Morphs it into a vessel. Half dead I forget Chronic. So I donate. Blood and skin to the Bipolar Genetics Repository. Bimonthly assessment forms to the Longitudinal Study. To help someone not born yet. Because there will be no cure for Chronic in my lifetime. It is why I stash my rainy-day-death-toll of pills that will change Chronic to Terminal. When Whitecoat won't discharge me until they are disposed of, I respond, "So, you've found a cure."

Mad Flora and Fauna Catalog: Kudzu

Kudzu is the chronic plant. It strangles out the foliage: soul crushers! And thrives. And multiplies. Spreads like neurotransmitter fuck ups that run patterns into the brain. Kudzu takes over until no one remembers what the landscape looked like, and there is no viable way back but to alter aesthetics. Call this transplanted heart and gills beautiful or at least enough. Figure out how to eat the leaves and make a cookbook where poison tastes good.

The Murderer: Primetime

I sit in my La-Z-Boy and watch myself on the 6 o'clock news. My fifteen minutes. Bagged Kate Spade and Anthony Bourdain. My work is put under the microscopes of cultural critics. I don't pay much attention—career hazard to see the impact to those left behind. Switch to *True Detective* on Netflix and pop a craft ale.

There is still my nemesis. She doesn't need me anymore, doesn't want me, stopped calling. Hell, I rarely flit across her brain after being her sole obsession for years. But I know where she lives in her new house with her wife and her dog. Track her successes on social media. She didn't friend me on Facebook, but I have other methods. I still plan to finish the job. Don't like the undone feel. Wakes me up some nights. And, yes, I know I'm supposed to focus on the larger picture. I've been privy to enough therapy sessions that I'm hip to the cognitive all-or-nothing trap. Can keep a gratitude journal until my smile freezes.

This was an unusual high profile week so I'm on the down low. I'll stay in this den and make strategic moves from the computer. So many of these pitifuls are already brink and nearly over—no skill involved—just an anonymous bully tweet. The workload is 24/7. Not just around holidays or full moons or in the spring anymore. I've quit my day job as an Eli Lilly drug rep (though similar skills and often the same results). And the young ones—I almost feel a pang for those teens—OD or brain all over from the family gun. I send a regular check to the NRA for making my job easy.

She haunts me—the one who slow danced in my grip. I'll wait. In the meantime, I've got several jumpers tonight, barely need to give them a nudge. An inept psychiatrist who just prescribed a 90 day supply of Ambien—call that done. And the suicide helpline with a fresh batch of volunteers. I still do my workouts at the local gym, keep my AR-15 oiled and ready. I have to be prepared for when she calls. Can't get lazy while the world is in apocalypse mode. Climate change, disillusionment, makes my job cake. Call it contract labor, call it an exit service. Evidence-based. Look at the stats. Tenth leading killer in the US. Had to chuckle to myself. Made the top ten list.

Temple

touch confident   she strokes my skull in gentle massage   ground
firm   breeze
on skin   birdsong soundtrack   better than muscle relaxants   in
ancient times
the ones who seized   seers   direct line to spirit   gods   prophecy
I get lost

temporal lobes   parietal lines   occipital gateway

going to the post office   forget the names of old friends   I ask
my love to place her fingertips where the current went in
through black batons to a relay I won't win   smooth
away   jostle of cells   & numb   gasp   reflex for air   strangers' prints
swallows dive &   storm   cast precursor winds   some kind of spell   I
wait
to break

The accumulation of days like the severe weather warning blaring airstream and media. A foot of snow an hour is hard to manage. It overtakes. Whites out space. I keep having severe weather warnings. They've become weather instead of events.

I develop pain in my right big toe joint. Attribute it to the seizures, all movement concentrated in the foot cuffed so the anesthesia and muscle relaxants didn't get there. It was awake for every session. It soothes me now that there was at least foot consciousness, my experiences registered by a body extremity. I connect my inability to relevé and the intense pain in my joint to the involuntary movements. Alternatively, I imagine someone getting in the way of my foot's dance in the closet-sized room, an injury unconscious to me. Now, even six years later, I often wake in the morning still in half sleep and my feet flutter, independent. Like they are working it out. Or regretful they couldn't just run the rest of my body out of there. Or like the spastic jerk moves of a hanged person's feet.

The Murderer: Murder Defense

I need to make my case. She edits my entries and twists my story to make it fit her survival. I'm a good guy. Not a stalker. Not creepy. She is like one of those breakups where the person says I never liked you to begin with. But she loved me. Wanted the whole package. *She* pursued *me*. Woke me up at all hours. Crisis calls as if I was 911 when my work calls for the coroner, not CPR. She told me I was her last hope, back-pocket plan. How is that supposed to make a guy feel? I just tried to meet her needs. Held quick on the roller coaster ride she took me on. In and out of locked hospital wards where she never put me on the visitor list. I worried. Binge-watched *Hinterland*. Took up smoking again. Chewed my nails to the quick. Eventually, she'd be out. Then apology texts. Would I meet for coffee? Forgive her? Even for a job a guy has limits. What I'm trying to say is I put up with a lot. Stayed steady. Kept her in my sights. Didn't waver in my commitment or resolve. There for her. Still.

Dear Murderer,

This is my goodbye sonnet. Fourteen lines and I'm out
of here. Alive! You try and detain me. Haunt my family. Sights
on my mother. She already in hospital. You, relentless. I block your attempts
with my survivor body on firmer ground than our last standoff. Remind you,
I won. Dare you to try and take her. Remind you of my reckless hurl into
hell, our contest of wills with mine nearly lost. Remind you of a curved form,
soft. Warn you, take advantage of the woman that birthed me and raised me
and loved me through all of your antics. I'll say it clearly:

I'll kill you.

With my own hands that would be yours, Murderer.
If you want me, you had your chance. Over and over
I was fair game. Repeat offender.
Psych system ingrate. You failed. Deal with it.

There is nothing for you here.

White Wedding

I'm fitted in a gaudy wedding dress all
sparkle
& twirl
& white.
Outfitted for the casket the crematorium.

        Little crows gather with their attraction to bling.

        Murderer employs a murder to nip at my seams.

Undo the glint.
Make the shine ragged threads.
Unravel the carapace.
Warp and weft.
Beak marks on shoulder blades rip bodice,

                              there goes what happened yesterday.
Talons etch my scalp destroy the veil,
                    there goes a moment from five years ago.
Sequin gone,
                                        there goes a name a face.
Epidermis chafes in rebuke.
The forgotten makes a constant itch, tight wool against breast.
He knew they'd pick me bare.

    Line their nests with long term and short term losses.

I'm still red-faced and blurry, but I can repeat things, like my name and *yes*. This constitutes that it is safe for me to leave. I insist on walking the aisle. He wants to carry me. Limp torso, legs sprawling out of the gown. No witnesses but the crows. Whitecoats have signed a disclaimer that they don't exist and nothing they do causes harm. I've signed a waiver to absolve them of liability. Murderer wrote the vows.

The crows gather on telephone lines awaiting the exchange of rings.

Diamonds! Diamonds! they croon.

Murderer produces a noose. Pronouncement from the DSM-V.

The crows caw.

DO YOU HAVE A LIVING WILL?

[*Written on the inside of the napkin accompanying the dinner trays for psych unit patients admitted for ECT treatment. Located in the inpatient discharge folder thanks to a mental health worker double agent working for ETC. THE RESISTANCE. Placed behind the safety plan worksheet that is not safe.*]

READ THIS IN PRIVATE. SHARE WITH OTHER INMATES CAREFUL TO NOT ALERT THE KEEPERS OR THE SHOCK BRIGADE

If you are receiving this note, you are in dire circumstances. Last ditch effort, any measures to keep you here. No doubt the "treatment" you are scheduled for has been touted as extremely effective with unbelievable success rates. They are unbelievable for a reason. Perhaps you watched the propaganda video with the soft colors & spa-like ambience—more luxury vacation than let's shoot kilowatts through your brain & hope for the best. No doubt they reassured you the memory loss is just around the time of treatment; the side effect of long term memory loss flashed on the screen for less than a second & not spoken out loud. You are told this is your best bet. Your loved ones, at a loss for what to do, jump on board because the ones with the white coats & MD by their names know best.

RUN. Get up out of the gurney & get the hell out. NOW. Slip your wristband off & make like a normate out of there. You may be like I was—indifferent, deathwish-ridden, an easy consent signature. Take my word. Take my body. Better, take my mind as amnesiac evidence. LEAVE. Tell them you ate food, which will buy you time. Retract your consent. If you are involuntary or a minor, we are coming to get you. At the bottom of this page is a contact. We are waiting for you. We are a tuned network nimble to alternative options, focused on thrive rather than survive, resourced & ready to receive you.

ETC. THE RESISTANCE

Testament

I am a cutter.

A killer.

A pill taker.

I am a high risk profile.

An easy target.

I am a wonder.

A still life version of survival.

I am a hoarder of insults.

An instrument of goodwill.

A fully manufactured human in broad daylight.

I am a miracle.

A walk thru rain water honest to god success story.

I am a lock up.

A throw away the keys 72-hour hold castaway.

I am a dry erase board name.

A walk-in ER case.

A DSM-V masterpiece.

I am an invisibility act complete with instructions.

A nightmare cast of characters.

A complex mess of neurotransmitters.

A backfired experiment.

I am a swollen eyed cry me a cure seeker.

I am a pusher.

A taker.

A shut up and listen session participator.

I am a wreck of scar muscle and infamy.

I am impulse and action.

I am hereditary predisposition and guilt.

I am a scale of 1 to 10.

I am diagnostic code 296.6.

A list of side effects and contraindications.

I am an IV.

A pumped stomach.

A hand overflowing.

I am stitch marks on inner right wrist.

I am a 911 call.

A pager number.

An unwritten note.

I am a neat appearance.

A perfect hello.

A well cut profile.

I am a shrink's hour.

A doctor's sidenote.

A wait-and-see game.

I am a wristband.

A siren.

A binder of paperwork.

I am an elegant signature.

A compliance to avoid sharp objects.

A real hard study.

I am a consent for treatment.

A repeat appearance.

A preventative measure.

I am a performer.

A crowdpleaser.

A light in the aftermath.

I am an attempt.

A statistic.

A permanent record of failure.

I am transcranial magnetic stimulation.

I am electroconvulsive therapy.

I am ketamine infusions.

I am a second chance, a third, a fourth.

A downward spiral.

An ultra-radian cycler.

I am hypomania in action.

I am   Zoloft

          Prozac

          Wellbutrin

Effexor

Risperdal

Parnate

Nortriptyline

Mirtazapine

Viibryd

Lexapro

Pristiq.

I am   Tegretol

Verapamil

Lithium

Neurontin

Depakote

Lamictal

Nimodipine

Trileptal.

I am   Zyprexa

Klonopin

Trilafon

Dexedrine

Seroquel

Geodon

Saphris

Abilify

Ativan.

I am 120 mg 3x/day.

I am use as directed.

I am take with food and

Do not operate heavy machinery.

I am a $1000 a day hospital bill.

I am a risk.

I am a hard sell.

Treatment resistant.

Impatient patient.

I am a high functioner.

A CYP2D6 Genotype ultrarapid metabolizer.

A mixed state.

A clean sell.

An insurance company's worst nightmare.

I am a once a week check-up.

A lockbox of potentials.

A prescription number.

A real shame.

A wasted talent.

I am an educator of corrosive content.

I am a dayroom unbreakable windowpane.

I am a quiet room.

I am under observation.

I am a voluntary/involuntary admittance.

I am the longest day.

I am a 15 minute SP check.

A low blood pressure read.

I am "the tulips are too excitable, it is winter here."

I am a lineage of insanity.

I am car exhaust.

Razor blades.

Temporary precautions.

I am a missing line.

A fake smile.

An I'm fine.

A subtle remainder.

I am a safety plan.

An educational DVD.

A confidentiality clause.

A garage door closing.

I am a drug tested on Himalayan rabbits.

I am   May

           Cause

           Nausea

           and

           Vomiting

           Constipation

           Dry

           Mouth.

I am   Shaking

            Hands

            Low

            Sex

            Drive

            Akathasia.

I am   Tachycardia

            Acne

            Weight

            Gain

            Somnolence.

I am   Increased

            Urination

            Cognitive

            Distortion

            Metallic

            Taste

            in

            Mouth.

I am a tainted gene pool.

I am the buck stops here.

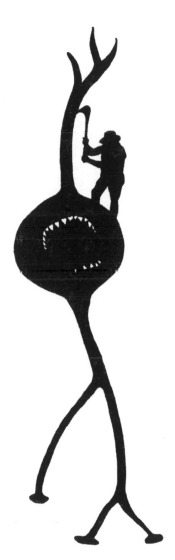

FIELD
NOTES

Jargon Translator

AC: Accessory Cephalic vein located in the forearm

DSM: Diagnostic and Statistical Manual of Mental Disorders

EBL: Estimated Blood Loss

ECT: Electroconvulsive Therapy

MRI: Magnetic Resonance Imaging

NPO: *Nil Per Os*, Latin for "nothing by mouth"

PICC: Peripherally Inserted Central Catheter

SP: Suicide Precautions

Notes

This book is informed by my lifelong experience with neurodiversity and mental health difference. I am bipolar and my daily life embraces changing bodymind states and shifting capacities. *Psych Murders* focuses on a five-year period between 2009 and 2014 when I experienced extreme mind states and suicidal ideation. During this time, I had over a dozen psych hospitalizations and medical treatments ranging from med trials to transcranial magnetic stimulation to shock to ketamine infusions.

It is imperative to mark the inherent racism, inequity, and disparity in the US health care system. As a white cisgender woman (also queer and disabled) with adequate health insurance and a supportive family, I was able to access treatments, therapies, and hospitals that are not available to everyone.

The poems in "Waiting Bay," "Treatment Room," and "Recovery Bay" are written from my personal experiences of electroshocks. The section titles are taken from terminology used by medical staff to refer to the curtained-off locations in a large space in the basement of the University Hospital, where ECT is conducted every weekday morning. *Index Series* is the term used in shock land to describe the initial 6–12 electroshocks that generally do the trick. Then there is *continuation* and *maintenance*. My course (or their course, depending) was approximately 30 sessions from October 2011 through March 2012.

The words in italics in "Procedure Details" are quotes from my psychiatry medical notes.

The "Mad Flora and Fauna Catalog" poems were written in response to interview questions from Ellen Redbird for a disability writing project.

"The Classifieds: Bipolar Girls on a Manic High are my Addiction" was inspired by the paper presentation "Deviant Sexuality and Disability: The Hypersexualization of Women with Bipolar Disorder" by Meghan O'Leary and Hallee Gibbons. Their talk was part of the Breaking Silences, Demanding Crip Justice: Sex, Sexuality, and Disability Conference at Wright State University in 2015.

"Temple" is dedicated to my wife, Petra Kuppers. This poem was written after a collaborative somatic and experiential anatomy exploration of the skull. We were gratefully harbored in fall mountain sunshine at Hambidge Center Artist Residency while waiting out Hurricane Matthew.

The sonnet "Dear Murderer" is after Terrance Hayes.

The cover art by Chanika Svetvilas is part of a drawing series, "What I have learned. (Fill in the blank.)" created during the coronavirus pandemic in 2020 with charcoal and collage on elementary school lined paper, 36 inches x 24 inches. The bipolar neuron in this piece is anthropomorphized as a reflection of her own mental health difference and challenges. She uses charcoal in her drawings as a transformative material whose activated form absorbs chemical substances, such as when a stomach is pumped after a medication overdose. Chanika Svetvilas is a Thai American interdisciplinary artist who utilizes lived experience as a way to interrogate psychiatric forms of care, create safe spaces, disrupt stereotypes, and reflect on contemporary issues as a cultural worker. www.chanikasvetvilas.com

Acknowledgments

Grateful celebration of the editors and publishers of these journals and anthologies in which this work has appeared, sometimes in different forms:

Anomaly: "Window Dressing"

Bombay Gin: "Forecast"

Disability Studies Quarterly: "Testament"

The Ending Hasn't Happened Yet: "Secondary Crime Scene"

In Corpore Sano: excerpts from "Waiting Bay," "Treatment Room," "Recovery Bay"

Pigment Extracted from the Past / It Never Dries: an anthology of self-elegies and essays: "The Murderer: Murder Defense, Primetime, 401K"

Rogue Agent: "(in)voluntary"

We Are Not Your Metaphor: "Neuromodulation Master," "ETC. The Resistance," excerpts from "Waiting Bay," "Treatment Room," "Recovery Bay"

Wordgathering: "Mad Flora and Fauna Catalog: Turtle"

Zoeglossia Poem of the Week: "Solar Eclipse," "Mad Flora and Fauna Catalog: Hyena, Kudzu"

Gratitude

I write these lines of gratitude on the autumn equinox, a day of equal light and equal dark. This afternoon I walked along Lake Michigan on my favorite beach in Benzie County. As I write this, Crystal Lake is alive with wavesong outside the window.

I want to acknowledge with deep respect the lands and waters that have held me during the writing of this book and their Indigenous past and present stewards: the Anishinaabe people—the Odawa and Ojibwe of Up North Michigan, and the Odawa, Ojibwe, and Potawatomi of what is colonially referred to as Ypsilanti, Michigan.

I also want to thank the beautiful web of people and places who have supported me in the making of this book—through writing and artistic exchange, classroom visit invitations, publication support, creative engagement. I offer deep thanks to all who helped me navigate (and continue to navigate) the lived experience this book holds:

To my parents, Judy and Roger Heit, to whom this book is dedicated. For their tenacity and resilience in bearing witness and supporting me during an impossible time, giving me shelter in multiple ways, changing their lives to accommodate my many treatments and hospitalizations, and for all of their love.

Brooke Wear, who gifted me the shock replacement term "my electrical work." Claudia F. Savage, who insisted I was still a poet even when I couldn't read or write. Barbara Dilley, who reminded me that I am an artist in a phone conversation after I finished ECT. Debra Horowitz, Joanna Preucel,

Gabrielle Edison: longtime friends and artists. Bill Scheffel (in memory), Stefanie Cohen, Denise Leto, Naomi Ortiz, Sophia Galifianakis, Vidhu Aggarwal, Megan Kaminski, TC Tolbert, Eleni Stecopoulos, Roxanna Bennett, Elæ Moss, Syrus Marcus Ware, Hannah Soyer, Raymond Luczak, Ally Day, Christine Neufeld, Liat Ben-Moshe, Dean Adams.

Gratitude also for my Zoeglossia family of disabled poets: my inaugural fellow cohort; founders Sheila Black, Jennifer Bartlett, and Connie Voisine; faculty Cecil Giscombe, Ellen McGrath Smith, and Ilya Kaminsky; and Meg Day, for the invaluable manuscript consultation and support.

To all the people who participated in The Asylum Project directed by Petra Kuppers and me as part of the Olimpias, an international disability performance collective: especially Anna Hickey-Moody for the invitation, VK Preston, April Sizemore-Barber, and all the hosts and participants for their experiential engagement with asylum in multiple forms.

To the artists in the Somatics/Illness/Disability Seminar facilitated by Petra and me as part of the Poetics: (The Next) 25 Years Conference at SUNY Buffalo, especially Declan Gould, Christina Vega-Westhoff, Jay Besemer, Andrew Giles.

To the organizers and participants in the Disability Arts and Culture Symposium at Eastern Michigan University. Thank you, my dear fellow panelists Jessica Suzanne Stokes and Gaia Celeste Thomas for our collaborative creation of "Disability Poetics & Crip Webs."

To all the discoers of Turtle Disco, a somatic writing space grounded in disability culture that Petra and I run out of our living room. Thank you to all who took part in my weekly Contemplative Dance & Writing Practice where many of these pieces got their start: especially to regulars Beth Currans, Sarah Dean, Carla Harryman, Elena SV Flys, and Dusty Ghastin.

To the TV series *Grey's Anatomy* and all the films I watched at the Michigan and State Theaters in Ann Arbor that distracted me with other worlds when mine felt uninhabitable.

To all the people and organizations who create time and space for artists. Vandaler Forening in Oslo, Norway. The Thicket on Tolomato Island in Darien, Georgia. The Hambidge Center in Rabun Gap, Georgia (where Murderer made his first appearance). To Jamie Figueroa for the retreat time in Santa Fe, New Mexico. To Summer Rodman for beautiful company and repeat oceanside stays in Fort Pierce, Florida.

Thank you to Wayne State University Press for making this book a beautiful reality: Annie Martin, for belief in this work; Kristin Harpster, Carrie Teefey, Kristina Stonehill for realizing it in the world; Polly Rosenwaike for copyedits; Lindsey Cleworth for design. To my anonymous peer reviewers. To Chanika Svetvilas for her artwork and bipolar solidarity.

Finally, gratitude to my beloved Petra: wife, partner, and collaborator in art/life who once upon a time introduced me to disability culture and told me to look up Mad pride and the psychiatric system survivor movement. It is a daily gift to dance with you in all the waters.

About the Author

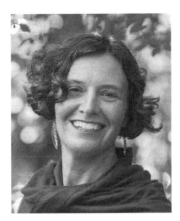

Photo by Tamara Wade

Stephanie Heit is a queer disabled poet, dancer, teacher, and codirector of Turtle Disco, a somatic writing space. She is a psych system/shock survivor, bipolar, a mad activist, Zoeglossia Fellow, and a member of Olimpias, a disability performance collective. She lives in Ypsilanti, Michigan, on Three Fires Confederacy territory and is the author of the poetry collection *The Color She Gave Gravity*.